NATURALLY
HEALED
the
HOLISTIC WAY:
A Comprehensive Guide

NATURALLY
HEALED
the
HOLISTIC WAY:
A Comprehensive Guide

LAKEISHA. M. DALE

XULON PRESS

Xulon Press
2301 Lucien Way #415
Maitland, FL 32751
407.339.4217
www.xulonpress.com

Unless otherwise indicated, Scripture quotations taken from the Holy Bible, New International Version (NIV). Copyright © 1973, 1978, 1984, 2011 by Biblica, Inc.™. Used by permission. All rights reserved.

Follow me on
YouTube Channel: Destine Living
Facebook: destine_living
Instagram: destine_living
Email: destine.living@gmail.com

Portrait Photo Credit
Photographer: Stephanie Mckinney
Stylist: Erica Joe

Paperback ISBN-13: 978-1-66281-507-2
Hard Cover ISBN-13: 978-1-66281-508-9
Ebook ISBN-13: 978-1-66281-509-6

I WANT TO FIRST DEDICATE THIS BOOK TO GOD who is the author and finisher of my faith. To my dedicated husband (Marco Dale), my supporter, and encourager. To my four children (Joel, Joseph, Josiah and Gracelyn), whom I love dearly. To my Parents: (Andre Jones and Linda Stampley Jones), thank you for being the godly example. To my siblings (Keith, Kendrick, Korey and Janiece) for your continued support. To my Aunts, Uncles and Cousins (too many to name) I will forever love you. Biological father (Keith) and stepmother. To my church family for trusting God in me to advise you on a better, healthier life, and last but not least, my pastors, Richard and Delmarie Stampley, and my spiritual parents (Mr. and Mrs. Marks), I love you!

DISCLAIMER

I AM NOT A MEDICAL DOCTOR. THE INFORMATION in this book is not intended or implied to be a substitute for professional medical advice, diagnosis, or treatment. All content, including text, graphics, images, and information contained in this book are for general information purposes only. I assume no responsibility for the accuracy of the information contained in this book. You are encouraged to confirm any information obtained from this book with your physician. Never disregard professional medical advice or delay seeking medical treatment because of something you have read in this book.

TABLE OF CONTENTS

My Personal Introduction Into Holistic Medicine

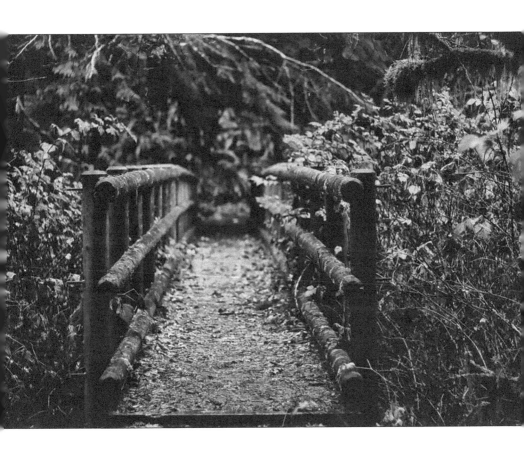

"But when he, the Spirit of truth, comes, he will guide you into all the truth. He will not speak on his own; he will speak only what he hears, and he will tell you what is yet to come." (John 16:13)

In 2019, my son began to have seizures; he was referred by his pediatrician to a specialist out of town. During this visit to the neurologist, he wanted us to start him on medicine that had outrageous side effects and wanted to put him to sleep to run tests. My husband and I refused the treatment and went home. As a parent I was caught between two realities; I did not want my son to continue to have seizures, but I did not want him on medication either. So, my husband and I did what we knew to do. We went on a 5-day consecration and prayed to God about what to do. During this time, the Holy Spirit told me that God had given us everything we need on earth; I just have to uncover the truth. (St. John 1: 3) "All things were made by him, and without him was not anything made that was made."

"And God said, see I have given you every herb that yields seed which is on the face of all the earth." (Genesis 1:29). As a result of this consecration, I made myself available to God and asked him to reveal the truth to me. I began studying what causes seizures and herbs that support the nervous system. I put my son on an herb that contains a mixture combination of elderberry and valerian root; to target his nervous system. I also put him on a children's probiotic to support his gut and digestion. Once starting him on the herbal regiment, he no longer had seizures. Within a year of my son's success, four other children with like stories contacted me and they also got on the same regimen as my son, and all of them have had nothing but positive results.

At the beginning of 2019, I was experiencing some pain and blood in my urine. I went to the emergency room twice. They gave me antibodies and it cleared up for about two weeks before it started again. Finally, they discovered I had kidney stones. I was referred to a Urologist. The doctor ran a test and discovered that I had three stones in total. Two stones were small enough to pass on their own, but the third would have to be broken up during a procedure. The procedure was canceled due to quarantining for COVID 19. During this time, I started searching for natural remedies to address kidney stones. I came across an herb called Chanca Piedra. I ordered the herb and started taking it with lemon water. Several months later, I was told by a Physician that not only did I only have one stone left, but that stone had shrunk to where it was passable. Staying away from starchy foods and food high in salt will also help with kidney stones.

My other children dealt with constant visits to the doctors' office due to allergies, asthma, ear infections, etc. I became tired of taking them to the doctor repeatedly, and giving them medicine that seemed to not work. I began to study herbs for my children and put them on a regimen that consists of elderberry, probiotics, and changed/added some things to their diet. Our biweekly visits to the pediatrician changed to a yearly wellness check. I remember taking one of my sons for his wellness check and upon arriving one of the medical assistants said to me, "Where y'all been, we haven't seen y'all in months. We were just talking about y'all the other day." My response to her was, "I took the holistic approach on y'all because I got tired of coming here and the medicine wasn't working." I then said to myself, that is a shame, the workers at the doctors' office knew us way too well. But my conversation with the worker at the doctors' office made me feel proud that my children were thriving healthily and confirmed to me that herbs work. Herbs provide healing for your whole body; therefore, herbs may take longer for effects to be recognized, but they do work.

Also, within this same year, my husband was rushed to the hospital one night. Upon arrival, it was discovered that his sugar was over 700. After staying a couple of nights at the hospital, my husband was diagnosed with diabetes and returned home with insulin. When he left the hospital his sugar levels were still in the mid 300 range. I begin studying herbs to give him. I started giving him cinnamon bark; cinnamon bark has many benefits but one of its benefits is to reduce blood sugar levels. We changed his diet and started him on an herbal regimen. My husband went for his two-week checkup and the doctor was amazed at how his sugar was lower; now in the lower 200 range. During his visit, he was told to monitor his blood pressure and continue to take insulin along with metformin. I began studying more natural remedies for diabetes and gained a better understanding of it. And began to search out answers to questions about the disease. If diabetes is a dietary disease, then why can't it be corrected through diet? The doctor said his pancreas gave out. What does the pancreas do? If the body was designed to make insulin why inject insulin instead of healing the body to do what it was designed to do by God? As I began to study the more knowledge I received about the disease. My husband went on a detox to purify his body of all impurities. He changed his diet and took away starch and sugars. I discovered that the pancreas produces insulin and works with the adrenal gland that helps to balance insulin in the body. So, I started giving him herbs that target these organs. Then I began to study the systems of the human body and realized that the pancreas is a part of the digestive system, so I began to give him herbs to target his whole digestive system. I started my husband on a weekly herbal regimen he was able to completely wean himself from all medicine and his sugar levels returned to normal. I gave him Flor de Manita.

As God gave me knowledge about the body and the functioning of it, I began to share information with friends and loved ones who all have personal testimonies about herbal health.

I felt God was pushing me into something I once never knew. Yes, I want to see people around me alive and healthy. As we live on this earth, I personally feel we should live it to the fullest in God and not be bent over sick and in pain. Some of the things shared in this book are things I studied and prayed about with family, friends, and loved ones concerning certain health conditions. There are many successful testimonies of the herbal benefits people around me received.

I decided to write this book to help others that may not have the time to study herbal benefits and the body. Information given in this book comes from knowledge given to me by God, searches online, articles read, personal experiences, etc.

This book is not an avenue or an excuse not to go to a physician. I personally go so I can get the specifics of what I need to work on within my body. I also will take the medicine to get immediate relief because I know medicine pacifies the symptoms (herbs work but can take a while to get into your system). Once getting the pain under control, I wean myself off the medicine and start herbal treatment because complete healing is my ultimate goal.

Holistic Approach
Verse Medicine

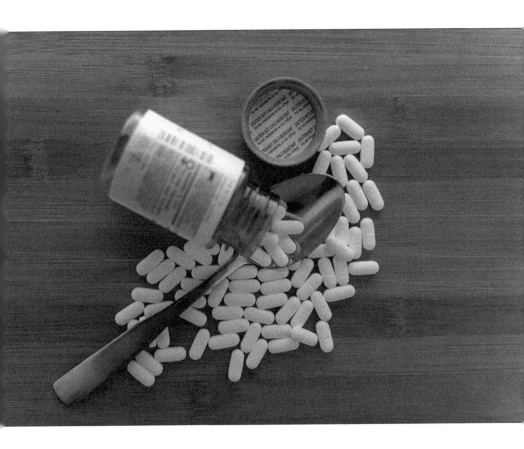

"In vain shalt thou use many medicines; for thou shalt
not be cured." (Jeremiah 46:11)

As I sat on the day and thought about the purpose of medicine, I realized that medicine pacifies the symptoms associated with the condition or disease, but never heals the root of the condition. An example of this is allergies or asthma; most medicine given will target and treat the runny nose, congestion, cough, or fever. Why not heal the lungs completely if it is asthma? Why not build the immune system so the body can have a strong defense against foreign substances?

My son was given an EpiPen for insect bites. I began to give him herbs to build his immune system. He has been bitten several times since I started building his immune system with herbs. He had an allergic reaction but nowhere near the point of needing an EpiPen.

I heard someone make a phenomenal statement, they said, "think about how many people you have heard die of medicine compared to how many people you have heard die-of herbs?" I realized that physicians are practicing medicine and it is my choice to choose the route best for me and my body. If you go to the doctor and receive medicine, and then go back because the first prescription did not work, your doctor will either up the dosage or try another type of medication; practicing medicine.

Probiotics instead of Antibodies

Probiotics help keep your body healthy and working well. They are made up of good bacteria. These bacteria fight off bad bacteria and help to support your immune system. Your gut contains roughly 70% of your immune system. Taking a probiotic daily will allow good bacteria to enter your gut, thus support and boost your immune system. Probiotics also aid in digestion support.

Whenever taking a strong antibiotic that causes diarrhea physicians usually advise you to take a probiotic to replace good bacteria in the body.

Antibodies neutralize and kill foreign bacteria and viruses. The more antibodies a person takes the more your body can become immune to it, causing antibody resistance, which is a growing problem. Yes, antibodies are needed for emergencies and the benefits of taking the antibody can outweigh the risks at given times. Antibodies were designed to neutralize and kill bad bacteria, infections, and diseases in the body. Be mindful that Antibodies can cause diarrhea, vomiting, etc. This can make the body extract good bacteria that the body needs.

In my cases antibiotics are necessary, please take them with caution, back it up with a probiotic. And drink plenty of water to flush your system. The body was designed to produce its own antibodies to fight against infection and disease. This can only happen when the immune system is healthy and strong. Taking a daily probiotic will aid your body with the capability to not only build your immune system but also make it strong enough to produce its own antibodies that will assist your body in fighting off sicknesses.

Essential Oils

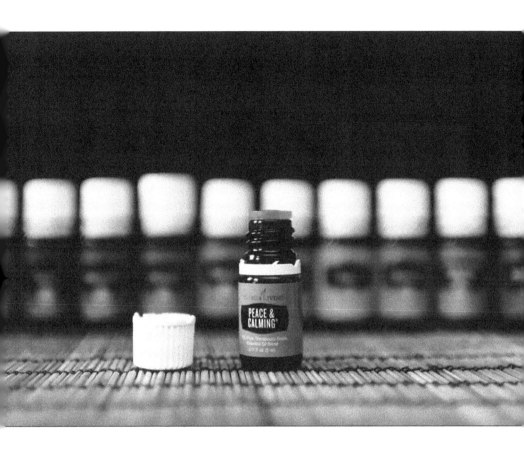

"And when they had opened their treasures, they presented gifts to Him: gold, frankincense, and myrrh" (Matthew 2:11).

"Is anyone among you sick? Let him call for the elders of the church, and let them pray over him, anointing him with oil in the name of the Lord. And the prayer of faith will save the one who is sick, and the Lord will raise him up." (James 5:14)

ESSENTIAL OIL IS A CHEMICAL COMPOUND FROM plants. Essential oils are known as the oil of the plant from which they were extracted, such as oil of clove, etc. The oils capture the plant's scent, and the unique aromatic oils are obtained through distillation, steam, and/or water.

Due to my personal experiences and my spiritual beliefs, one must be cautious of the oils burnt in your dwelling. Essential oils have many benefits. Burning incense can ward off spirits, invite the evil spirit, purify the surroundings and when inhaled can cause healing, by destroying bacteria, fungus, and viruses in the atmosphere and within your body. Research has shown that bacteria in the air can be reduced up to 94% by burning incense for an hour.

After doing much research and prayer, I discovered a particular faith-based company that I now buy my essential oils from.

Essential oils can reduce stress, anxiety, and aid sleep; for example, breathing in lavender oil. Essential oils can stimulate creativity by clearing and stimulating the mind. This method is used in yoga, and meditation practices. Essential oils can purify your space, Buddhist monks use them in this sense. These oils can trigger memories and boost moods. Rosemary, peppermint, and citrus oils can calm and improve focus and mental clarity.

Seven Oils mentioned in the Bible

#1:Cinnamon "Then the Lord said to Moses, Take the following fine spices: 500 shekels of liquid myrrh, half as much (that is, 250 shekels) of fragrant cinnamon, 250 shekels of fragrant calamus, 500 shekels of cassia—all according to the sanctuary shekel—and a hint of olive oil. Make these into a sacred anointing oil, a fragrant blend, the work of a perfumer. It will be the sacred anointing oil. Then use it to anoint the tent of meeting, the ark of the covenant law, the table and all its articles, the lampstand and its accessories, the altar of incense, the altar of burnt offering and all its utensils, and the basin with its stand." (Exodus 30:22-28).
Cinnamon can help with stomach ulcers, antiparasitic worms, digestive issues (apply 2-4 drops on your stomach), add to toothpaste, and soothe your throat (dissolve in hot tea.)

#2:Frankincense "And when they had opened their treasures, they presented gifts to Him: gold, frankincense, and myrrh." (Matthew 2:11).

Frankincense was used to heal any disease that plagued people during BC times.

Frankincense can be used to boost immunity, shrink tumors, and decrease inflammation.

#3:Hyssop "Purge me with hyssop, and I shall be clean; wash me, and I shall be whiter than snow." (Psalms 51:7).

Hyssop can be used to stimulate creativity and help open the circulatory system.

#4:Cedarwood: "The priest shall order that two live clean birds and some cedar wood, scarlet yarn and hyssop be brought for the person to be cleansed." (Leviticus 14:4).

Cedarwood oil can aid in sleeping, ADHD, and assist in hair loss.

#5 Balsam Fir: (oil taken from the fir tree) "Then David and all the house of Israel played music before the Lord on all kinds of instruments of fir wood, on harps, on stringed instruments, on tambourine, on sistrums, and on cymbals." (2samuel 6:5).

Balsam Fir can be used to heal throat and sinus infections, urinary tract infections, and arthritis.

#6 Myrtle: "Go out to the mountain, and bring olive branches, branches of oil trees, myrtle branches, palm branches, and branches of leafy trees, to make booths, as it is written." (Nehemiah 8:15).

Myrtle can be used for a variety of health benefits like soothing the respiratory system, balancing thyroids, etc.

#7 Myrrh: "On coming to the house, they saw the child with his mother Mary and bowed down and worshiped him. Then they opened their treasures and presented him with gifts of gold, frankincense, and myrrh." (Matthew 2:11).

Myrrh can control diabetes, aid in eczema, and ringworm.

[Michell S. Lazurek.] [7 Healing Oils Found in the Bible.] [9/7/20.] [www.biblestudytools.com/bible-study/topical-studies/healing-oils-found-in-the-bible.html.]

Index of Essential oils and benefits (A-Z)

Some of the oils listed below can be mixed with body cream (preferably shea butter) and applied to the body.

One of the most effective ways to benefit from essential oils is to put oil in a diffuser.

- Bergamot- regulate appetite (aid anorexia and obesity), antidepressant, insect repellant, etc.

- Cinnamon Bark- cough, colds, support a healthy immune system, support healthy metabolic function, etc.
- Cedarwood- acne, dandruff, eczema. Fungal infection, greasy skin, ulcers, bronchitis, congestion, nervous tension, stress relief, sleep-inducing, etc.
- Chamomile- helps relieve anxiety, mental clarity, etc.
- Clary Sage- helps fight bacteria in the digestive system, urinary tract, and excretory system, etc.
- Clove Bud- digestive health, helps with hiccups, indigestion, motion sickness, excess gas, relieves stress, helps lessen mental exhaustion, helps with depression, anxiety, and insomnia, etc.
- Coriander- aids in digestion, relaxation aches, pains, and arthritis.
- Cypress- fights infections, aids the respiratory system, removes toxins from the body, stimulates relief to the nerves, and helps with anxiety, etc.
- Eucalyptus-decongestion, anti-inflammatory properties can be used to address skin, ear, nose, and throat problems, urinary ailments, fever, and arthritis, etc.
- Fennel- can help with digestion, respiratory system, female reproductive system, detoxifier for excessive foods or alcohol, effective on bug bites when properly diluted, etc.
- Frankincense- skincare preparations for prevention of wrinkles, dry damaged or mature skin, supports the immune system, promotes nerve regeneration and improves the function of crushed nerves, depression,

decongestion, sacred uses, instills deep tranquility of the mind, can slow breathing rate (making it ideal for meditation purposes), etc.

- Geranium- aids in skincare, reproductive system, nervous system, lymphatic/endocrine system, an antiseptic, anti-inflammatory and detoxifies the body, relaxation and relieve tension, etc.
- Ginger- useful for digestive issues (indigestion, constipation, diarrhea, and nausea), a sexual tonic for impotence, chronic bronchitis, aid in circulatory stimulants to address cold hands and feet, cardiac fatigue, angina pectoris, muscle pain, joint pain, colds, flu, prevention of morning sickness in pregnancy, motion sickness, and nausea, etc.
- Grapefruit- suppresses appetite, promotes weight loss, helps balance mood, antibacterial, and antimicrobial effects, helps reduce stress and lower blood pressure, treats acne, cardiovascular support, etc.
- Helichrysum- arthritis, reduces scarring, heals wounds and burns, treats acne, etc.
- Ho Wood- (similar to Eucalyptus) promotes peace and tranquility, helps the mind relax, general pain, minor wounds, insect bites, colds, inflammation, etc.
- Juniper Berry- purges toxins from the body, increases urination to flush toxins from the body, clears urinary tract infections, cleanses the circulatory-lymphatic system, addresses swelling and cellulite, etc.
- Lavender- soothes burns, takes the sting out of insect bites, calms headaches, anxiety, promotes relaxation,

treats fungal infections, allergies, depression, insomnia, eczema, nausea, and menstrual cramps, etc.
- Lemon- helps lower fever, lifts the spirit, improves concentration and memory, boosts the immune system and strengthens circulation, etc.
- Lemongrass- helps with an underactive thyroid (use with Myrrh), helps digestive problems, high blood pressure, antibacterial, antifungal, and anti-inflammatory properties, helps to prevent gastric ulcers, relieve nausea and diarrhea, etc.
- Lime- helps treat internal infections, helps balance blood sugar, supports immune function, etc.
- Marjoram- used for nerves, heart, blood circulation, coughs, gall bladder, stomach cramps, digestive disorders, depression, dizziness, migraines, nervous headaches, nerve pain, paralysis, coughs, runny nose, etc.
- Myrrh- helps kill harmful bacteria, parasites, support oral health, helps heal skin sores and eases pain and swelling, etc.
- Orange- colds, constipation, digestion, flatulence, flu and stress, etc.
- Orange Blossom- reduce cortisol levels, lower blood pressure, improve menopause symptoms, reduce inflammation, anti-bacterial agent, rejuvenate the skin, stimulate cell growth, etc.
- Oregano- a natural antibiotic, helps lower cholesterol, help treat yeast infections, may improve gut health, help relieve pain, help cancer-fighting properties, have anti-inflammatory properties, etc.

- Palmarosa- support clean, healthy-looking skin as well as balance moisture levels in the skin, etc.
- Patchouli- treat skin conditions (acne, dry and cracked skin), ease colds, headaches, and upset stomach. Also relieves depression, provides relaxation, eases stress, and anxiety. It helps with oily hair, dandruff, and controls appetite,
- Peppermint- helps with headaches, migraines, PMS symptoms, digestive concerns, motion sickness, nausea, irritable colon, respiratory issues, liver tonic, insect repellent, etc.
- Pine- purifies and cleanses the air, clears negative energy, provides protective energy, etc.
- Rose- eases pain, relieves menstrual discomfort, decreases anxiety and stress, antibacterial, antifungal properties, stimulates sex drive, eases depressive symptoms, etc.
- Rosemary- may improve brain function, stimulate hair growth, help relieve pain, repel certain bugs, ease stress, increase circulation, help perk you up, reduce joint inflammation, etc.
- Sandalwood- heart health, heal scars, relax the mind and body (used by several pagan religions), etc.
- Spearmint- helps relieve headache, digestion problems, high in antioxidants, aids women with hormone imbalance, improves memory, fights bacterial infections, lowers blood sugar, helps to reduce stress, etc.

- Tea Tree- helps to fight germs, support and boost the immune system, fight infections, calms, can ease stress, etc.
- Turmeric- eliminates acne, fine lines, and wrinkles, blemishes, and marks (when used as a facial mask), get rid of dandruff, hair loss, and can treat scalp conditions.
- Vetiver- helps improve breathing pattern, relieve stress, emotional traumas, shock, lice, repel insects, arthritis, stings, and burns, relieves nervousness, insomnia, and joint and muscle pain, etc.
- Ylang Ylang- boosts mood, reduces depression, alleviates anxiety, lowers blood pressure, decreases heart rate, stimulates oil production in the skin and on the scalp, repels flying insects and kills bug larvae, stimulates the scalp and promotes fuller and thicker hair, etc.

Single Oils. (2020). Retrieved from https://www.byfaithoils.org/collections/essential-oils
[Emily Rekstis.] [Essential Oils 101: Finding the Right One for You.] [7/3/2018.] [https://www.healthline.com/health/essential-oils-find-the-right-one-for-you.]

ACUPRESSURE/
ACUPUNCTURE

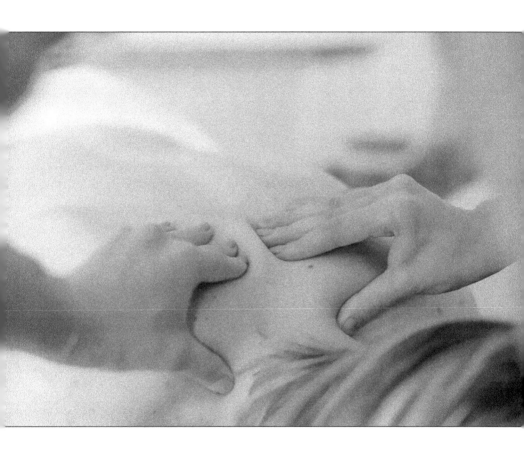

"Do not be anxious about anything, but in everything, by prayer and petition, with thanksgiving, present your requests to God. And the peace of God, which transcends all understanding, will guard your hearts and your minds in Christ Jesus." (Philippians 4:6-7)

ACUPUNCTURE- A SYSTEM OF INTEGRATIVE MED-
icine that involves pricking the skin or tissue with needles.
Used to alleviate pain and to treat various physical, mental,
and emotional conditions. Originated in ancient China.

Acupressure- the application of pressure (as with the
thumbs or fingertips) to certain points of the body to stimulate therapeutic effects (such as relief to tension or pain).
It releases muscular tension and promotes the circulation of
blood and the body's life force to aid healing.

Acupuncture can be achieved by needle puncture through
the skin. Acupressure can be achieved by using your fingers.
Acupressure can help with acne, eczema, other skin problems, allergies, ankle and foot problems, anxiety and nervousness, arthritis and non-articular rheumatism, asthma and
breathing difficulties, backache and sciatica, chronic fatigue
syndrome, colds and flu, constipation, cramps and spasms,
depression and emotional balancing, diarrhea, earaches, eye-
strain, fainting, hangovers, headaches and migraines, hiccups, hot flashes, immune system boosting, impotency and
sexual problems, insomnia, irritability, frustration, dealing
with change, jaw problems, knee pain, labor, delivery and
nursing, memory and concentration, menstrual tension,
cramps, and PMS, motion sickness, morning sickness, and
nausea, neck tension and pain, nosebleeds, pain, pregnancy
and infertility, shoulder tension, sinus problems and hay
fever, stomachaches, indigestion, and heartburn, swelling

and water retention, toothaches, wrist pain, carpal tunnel syndrome, and tendonitis.

Acupressure can help with relief and healing from various things.

Pressing on certain points of your body for a certain amount of time can aid in healing in all the areas listed above. A great book that describes and lists all acupressure points is called '*Acupressure's Potent Points*' by, Michael Reed Gach. I have used information from this book to relieve pain within my own body and it helped tremendously.

Gach, Michael Reed. (2009) *Acupressure's Potent Points. New York: New York*

Knowing the
Body Systems

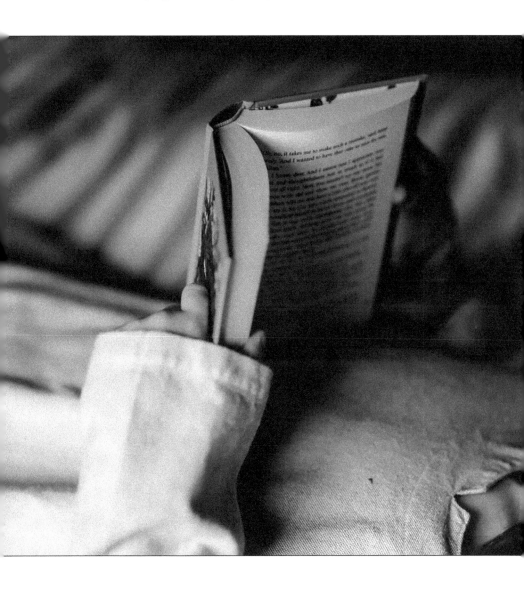

"*My people are destroyed for lack of knowledge: because thou hast rejected knowledge...*" (Hosea 4:6)

ONE DAY I WAS IN PRAYER ASKING GOD FOR understanding about the body and I could hear the Holy Spirit speak to me by saying that most of the time the body is sick due to a deficiency, or lack of something that can be replenished through diet, supplements, minerals, herbs, etc. One example of this may be dehydration; the body lacks enough liquid. I find this to be true to many sicknesses and diseases. It could be a lack of vitamin C, b12, etc. Sometimes our bodies can be sick because it possesses too much of something, like toxins, parasites, etc. I believe in God for total healing in every area of life. I also believe that the body was designed to heal itself, but it must be in shape to do so. There are things we can do on our part to be good stewards of our temple.

Having a good understanding of the body systems is key to successfully selecting the right herbs, supplements, or minerals for healing. An example of this is someone who may experience a cough or pain in their chest. Most people may say my chest is hurting or I cannot stop coughing. The pain or cough is just simply the symptom of an underlying issue. The pain or cough could be congestion by way of mucus built up in the lungs. Some people will begin treatment by targeting the lungs; the lungs are an organ. Instead of solely focusing on the symptoms of the sickness or on the organ that produces the symptoms, the main focus should be on the respiratory system. Focusing on the whole system instead of just an organ or symptoms (like medication tends to do), triggers immediate and complete healing. After selecting herbs that cater to the whole system, I would advise you to then select herbs that will heal the organ. Once selecting the right herb for both the system and the organ, I suggest starting a regimen for these herbs. For example, MWF consumes herbs for the system and T/Th/Sat consumes herbs for the targeted organ. If a person is already on modern medicine, I suggest weaning off the medicine for at least two weeks. This gives the herbs time to get into your system. Herbs work. They just take longer to get into your system compared to modern medicine. This is one of the reasons why I would also suggest taking a liquid form rather than capsules; despite the terrible taste of liquid herbs, there are major benefits. When taking capsules your body still must digest the product and sometimes your body will dispose of it in waste, making it less beneficial in some cases.

Below is a table of the eleven major systems and organs for the human body. This graph can be used to get a better understanding of your body as well as help you target where healing needs to begin.

Major Organ Systems

System	Organs in the System	Some Major Functions of the System
Cardiovascular	Heart, Blood Vessels (arteries, capillaries, veins)	Pumps blood and circulates it throughout the body

Respiratory	Nose, Mouth, Pharynx, Larynx, Trachea, Bronchi, Lungs	Add oxygen to the blood (and removes carbon dioxide from the blood)
Nervous	Brain, Spinal cord, Nerves (both those that carry impulses to the brain and those that carry impulses from the brain to muscles and organs)	Directs intentional (and many automatic) actions of the body. Enable thinking, self-awareness, and emotions
Skin	Skin (both the surface that is generally thought of as skin and the underlying structures of connective tissue, including fat, glands, and blood vessels)	Provides barrier protection between the inside of the body and the external environment
Musculoskeletal	Muscles, Tendons and Ligaments, Bones, Joints	Provides structure and allows motion of the body
Blood	Red blood cells, White blood cells, Platelets, Plasma (the liquid part of the blood), Bone Marrow (where blood cells are produced), Spleen, Thymus	Transports oxygen and nutrients to all the cells of the body (and removes carbon dioxide and waste products)
Digestive	Mouth, Esophagus, Stomach, Small Intestine, Large Intestine, Rectum, Anus, Liver, Gallbladder, Pancreas (the part that produces enzymes), Appendix	Extracts nutrients from foods excrete waste products from the body

Endocrine	Thyroid Gland, Parathyroid Gland, Adrenal Gland, Pituitary Gland, Pancreas (the part that produces insulin and other hormones), Stomach (the cells that produce gastrin), Pineal Gland, Ovaries, Testes	Produces chemical messengers carried in the blood, which directs the activities of different organ systems
Urinary	Kidney, Ureters, Bladder Urethra	Filters waste products from the blood
Male Reproductive	Penis, Prostate Gland, Seminal Vesicles, Vasa Deferentia, Testes	Enables reproduction
Female Reproductive	Vagina, Cervix, Uterus, Fallopian Tubes, Ovaries	Enables reproduction

[Merck Sharp & Dohme Corp.,] [Organ Systems.] [2020] [https://www.merckmanuals.com/home/fundamentals/the-human-body/organ-systems#v13391939]

GENERAL HEALTH

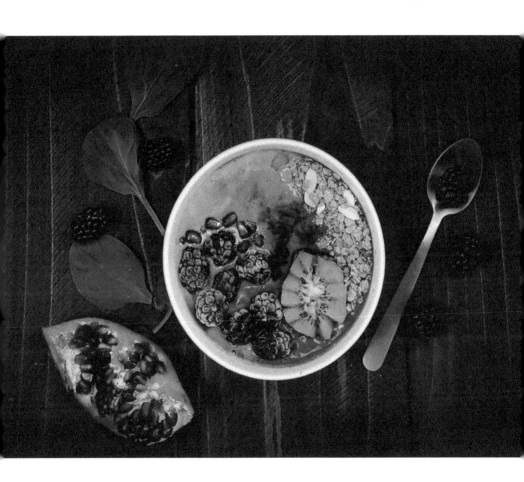

"Beloved, I pray that all may go well with you and that you may be in good health, as it goes well with your soul." (3 John 1:2)

UNDERSTANDING THE pH LEVEL OF THE HUMAN body is extremely important. An alkaline state body (pH level 7.1-14.0) produces a strong immune system, promotes weight loss, improves kidney health, prevents cancer, and prevents heart disease, etc. A pH level of 7.0 is a neutral body state. An Acidic state body (pH level of 0-6.9) makes the body accessible for disease and infection to thrive in.

Consuming a balanced diet will keep your body healthy and your immune system strong. If you are someone that eats a lot of acidic foods (like fish), consume some alkaline foods (like spinach) within the same meal to balance your diet. Personally, the closer you can get your body to a pH level of 14, the better.

Acidic foods are meat, poultry, fish, dairy, eggs, and grains. Neutral foods are natural fats, starches, and sugars. Alkaline foods are fruits, nuts, legumes, and vegetables. [https://www.healthline.com/nutrition/the-alkaline-diet-myth.]

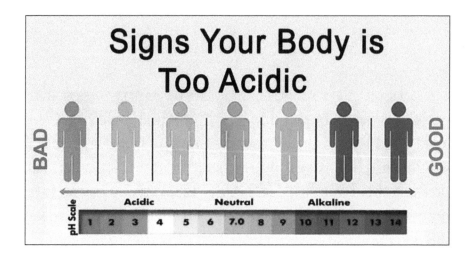

[Tr growth / Shutterstock.] [pH in the Human Body.] [Aug 24, 2018.] [https://www.news-medical.net/health/pH-in-the-Human-Body.aspx.]

As with any sickness, disease, cold, or flu, the key is to build your immune system. Some key things I have found to do are vitamin c and zinc. Sodium Ascorbate vitamin c is an outstanding form of vitamin c and is highly recommended.

More General Health Tips

1. Drink plenty of water daily (preferably 1 gallon a day), water helps keep your body flushed from impurities and toxins.
2. Aim to eat a plant-based diet.
3. When eating chew food thoroughly before swallowing. This may seem silly to some people, but once while I was eating, I could hear God speak to my spirit saying,

notice the size of the food you swallow. I realized immediately that I do not chew my food thoroughly before swallowing. Then I could hear God tell me that when you do this you cause more work for your digestive system to break down the food and make it more susceptible for you to clog the digestive system, stomach, and gut. Food should be like mush before swallowing, never swallow food in chunks.

4. This may be hard for some people but try not to drink while eating; this too can cause blockage in your digestive system. This can slow the digestive process down by causing the stomach to be acidic and can water down the natural juices of the stomach. After eating try to wait at least 30 mins to an hour before consuming a beverage. This will cause your food to start the digestive process.

5. When researching things to eat, drink, or take look for things that have a multi-beneficial purpose like CBD. CBD comes from a hemp plant, relieves pain, stress, anxiety, reduces blood sugar levels, etc.

6. A healthy gut is a healthy person. As stated previously, a large percentage of the immune system is in the gut. Keep your gut clean and flushed from toxins and unnecessary build-up.

7. Most people are asleep, on their way to work, or just simply inside during the sunrise. God has so many healing incentives attached to the sun rays; being outside during the sunrise, can naturally boost your energy,

metabolism, and some glands. Some scientists believe that the sun possesses the key to optimal health.

8. Viruses, wash hands with soap and water. Viruses enter the body through the mouth, nose, and ears. Doing an alcohol rub around these three areas will prevent viruses from entering the body.

If you choose to take medication with herbs, take herbs 2 hours before or after medication; this a good way to wean the body from medication.

9. When you wake up in the morning, consume warm liquid (warm water or decaffeinated tea) this will cleanse digestion and help flush out toxins and soothe the digestive tract and make it easier to get rid of waste from the day before and help with digestion for the rest of the day. This also reduces stress, circulation, and weight loss.

10. Great general everyday herbs to consume is vitamin c, Zinc, and Elderberry. Herbs are powerful for simply building the immune system

11. Be a label reader; read the ingredient label of every-thing you consume. Monitor what you put in your body. Things to monitor are white sugar, sodium, car-bohydrates, and calories.

Recommended detox and cleansers

There are so many detoxes and cleansers available. I personally strictly stick to detoxes that cleanse more than one area of the body. I try to target as many systems as possible at one time. It is good to do a full body detox quarterly to cleanse your body from toxins and undigested food. When consuming food, some food is digested and fueled by the body for energy, function, and productivity. Some of the food is deposited for waste and your body discards it. But what happens to the food that is neither digested nor excreted from the body? It builds up in your body and organs, which leaves room for sickness, infection, and diseases.

Another reason to detox your body regularly is that detoxing can start the healing process. If you consider using herbs to heal your body, boost your immune system, or help with staying healthy, it is always good to flush your body from all impurities before starting. This gives the herbs a clean slate to begin the healing process. Starting herbs without detoxing the body first can prolong the healing process because the herbs have to penetrate through all the pre-existing bad stuff in the body.

Doing a blood cleanse is another form of detox. The blood carries oxygen and trillions of cells to all the organs of your body and if the body has toxins in the blood these toxins will enter the lungs, liver, and kidneys. The blood must flow and function clean, clear, and without any interruptions. For people that have high blood pressure, diabetes, and cholesterol issues, I usually recommend they do a blood cleaner 1st before starting herbs.

What are herbs?

Herbs are any leaves, seeds, or flowers used for flavoring, food, medicine, or perfume.

"And God said, "let the earth bring forth grass, the herb yielding seed, and the fruit tree yielding fruit after his kind, whose seed is in itself, upon the earth: and it was so." (Genesis 1:11).

The awesome thing about God is not only was the body designed to heal itself, but God has given us everything we need in the earth realm for us to be healthy vibrant beings.

Benefits of Nutmeg

Helps relieve pain, increases immune system function, can prevent leukemia, improve blood circulation, soothe indigestion, strengthen cognitive function, detoxify the body, boost skin health, alleviate oral conditions, and reduce insomnia.

Benefits of lemon and water

I like to call this fruit the golden fruit.

Consuming lemon and water can help to reduce acid reflux, fever, dissolve and prevent kidney stones, help with a sore throat, lymph nodes, keep colon digestion clean, promote weight loss, prevent cancer, prevent heart disease, and contains vitamin c.

Lemon is acidic outside the body, but once it is fully digested in the body, it puts the body in an alkaline state, which will boost the immune system.

Benefits of CBD
Relieves anxiety, stress, physical discomfort, improves focus, creativity, insomnia, and provides feelings of tranquility and peace.

Hemp Seed Oil
Nourishes the heart and circulatory system, regulates cholesterol, helps boost mood, balance emotions and support restful sleep. Reduces risks of Alzheimer's disease and reduces inflammation in the body.

Benefits of Coconut Oil
comes in many forms, capsules, liquid, and soft gels.

Provides healthy skin, nails, weight loss, hair growth, supports cardiovascular and brain health, energy levels and also helps with constipation.

Benefits of White Oak Bark
Used for arthritis, diarrhea, colds, fever, cough, and bronchitis. Stimulates appetite and improves digestion.

Benefits of Red Palm Oil
Reduces cholesterol levels, slows the progression of heart disease, boosts brain health, enhances vitamin A, reduces stress, and improves skin and hair health.

Benefits of Elderberry

Helps in weight loss, boosts the immune system, reduces the appearance of wrinkles and age spots, aids in eliminating excess cholesterol from the body, promotes bone strength and development of new bone tissue, alleviates respiratory conditions such as cold and cough, eliminates constipation and boosts the digestive system, reduces blood pressure and aids in managing diabetes.

Benefits of Papaya

Build blood platelets, fights cancer, provides strength to the body, protects arthritis, decreases the risk of cataracts, helps the rebuilding of muscle and its tissue, helps you lose weight, relieves toothaches, boosts digestive health, regulates the menstrual cycle, improves immunity and heart health, reduces acne and burns, treats eye health, fights against intestinal worms, keeps skin glowing and smooth and flattens the stomach.

Benefits of Apple Cider Vinegar

Natural laxative, improves digestion, lowers blood sugar levels, improves insulin sensitivity, helps to lose weight, reduce belly fat, lower cholesterol, lowers blood pressure, improves hair health, anti-aging properties, makes you feel fuller, helps reduce acne, reduces bloating, aids heartburn, decreases cancer risks, kills bacteria, contains antioxidants and is also good for heart health.

Benefits of Turmeric

Prevents heart disease, eye conditions, and Alzheimer's, has anti-inflammatory properties, helps with arthritis, reduces the risk of spreading cancer.

Benefits of Kombucha Tea

Source of probiotics, kills bacteria, reduces heart disease, helps manage type 2 diabetes, may also help protect against cancer.

Benefits of White Willow

This herb is a natural aspirin, can be used to relieve menstrual cramps, bring down a fever, inflammation, and pain.

Benefits of Wheat Plant

May reduce cholesterol, help kill cancer cells, aid in blood sugar regulation, can alleviate inflammation, and help promote weight loss.

Benefits of Echinacea Plant

Boost the immune system (fight against germs), increases the number of white blood cells (fight against infections).

Benefits of Lilly of the Valley

Used for heart problems, urinary tract infections, kidney stones, weak contractions in labor, epilepsy, fluid retention, strokes, paralysis, eye infections, and leprosy.

Benefits of Prickly Ash Bark

Used for menstrual cramps, blood circulation problems in the legs and fingers, joint pain, toothaches, sores, to also break a fever and treat ulcers.

Benefits of Black Seed Oil

Treat asthma, skin conditions, lower blood sugar and cholesterol levels, aid in weight loss, and protect brain health.

Cooking Oil:

Cook with oils that do not clog your arteries. Suggested oils are grapeseed oil, sesame oil, hemp seed oil, or avocado oil.

HERBAL SUPPORT (A-Z)

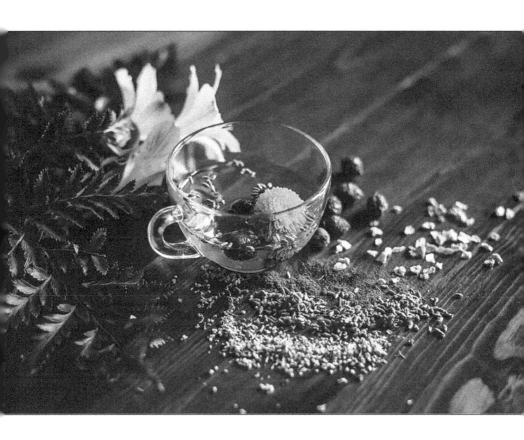

"The Lord sustains him on his sickbed; in his illness, you restore him to full health." (Psalms 41:3)

MANY HERBALISTS OUT THERE SUGGEST TAKING this list of herbs below and search herbalist that offer them.

Consume herbs in tea, smoothies, and or natural juices.

The human body has eleven systems, listed below are suggested herbs that can be used to help support and help improve each body systems and ultimately aid in healing. Be mindful that this is only a shortlist, numerous herbs that will benefit each system.

1. **Circulatory System (circulate blood throughout the body)-** Hawthorn Berry Syrup, Cayenne Pepper, Eleuthero Root, Garlic, Ginger Root, Goldenseal Root, and Parsley. Additional herbs are Iron, Vitamin B, Bacopa, Chickweed, and Maidenhair.

2. **Digestive System (absorb nutrients and remove waste)-** Sea moss, Bladderwrack, Slippery Elm Bark, and Licorice Root. Additional Herbs are Yellow Dock Root, Burdock Root, and Cocolmeca.

3. **Endocrine System (hormones)-** Black Cohosh Root, Sarsaparilla Root, American Ginseng Root, Licorice Root. Additional things, False Unicorn Root, Blessed Thistle Herb, Squaw Vine Herb, Avocados, Hemp Seeds, Walnuts, and Green Leafy Vegetables.

4. **Integumentary System (skin, hair, nails, sweat, glands)-** Queen Anne's Lace Herb, Gotu Kola Herb,

Ginkgo Leaf, Mullein Leaf, Oregon Grape Root. Lobelia Herb, American Ginseng Root.

5. **Lymphatic/Immune System (defends the body against pathogens)-** Astragalus Root, Eleuthero Root, Echinacea Purpure Root, Echinacea Purpurea Herb, and Reishi Mushroom

6. **Muscular System (allows the body to move)-** Chamomile, Turmeric, Cinnamon, Ginger, and CatsClaw.

7. **Nervous System (process information to the brain)-** Valerian Root, Elderberry, Coconut Oil, Skullcap Herb, Oregon Grape Root, St. John's Wort Herb.

8. **Reproductive System (produce offspring)-**
   a. **Male- Sarsaparilla, Yohimbe, Locust Bark, Capadulla, and Irish Sea m\Moss**
   b. **Female- Hydrangea, Damiana, Sarsaparilla, and Sea Moss**

9. **Respiratory System (bring air in and out of the lungs)-** Nettle Leaf, Mullein Leaf, Fresh Garlic, Fennel Seed & Chickweed Herb.

10. **Skeletal System (bones)-**
    White Oak Bark, Lungwort Herb, Marshmallow Root, Mullein Leaf, Black Walnut Leaf, Gravel Root, Slippery Elm Bark, Wormwood Herb, Plantain Leaf, Lobelia Herb, Skullcap Herb & Aloe Vera Gel Powder 100:1

11. **Urinary/Excretory System (filter blood to produce urine and get rid of waste)-** Goldenrod (Solidago Canadensis), Corn Silk, Horsetail Herb, Uva-Ursi Leaf, Juniper Berry.

The human body has a total of 78 organs. Some organs and suggested herbs are listed below, these suggested herbs can be used to help support and improve each organ and ultimately aid in healing (the first 3-5 herbs listed are the most beneficial). Next to each organ is a number given, this organ correlates to the system in which the organ dwells in.

Adrenal Gland-3- Mullein Leaf, Licorice Root, Eleuthero Root, Gotu Kola Herb, Hawthorn Berry, Lobelia Herb, Ginger Root, and Cayenne Root.

Arteries- 1- Hawthorn Berry Juice Concentrate, and Pure Vegetable Glycerin

Bladder-11- Bladderwrack, Black Cohosh Root, Ginger Root, Gravel Root, Juniper Berry, Lobelia Herb, Marshmallow Root, Parsley Root, Uva-Ursi Leaf, and White Pond Lily.

Bones-10- Horsetail, and Arnica Montana.

Bone Marrow-5- TSY-1 (Tianshengyuan-1)

Brain-7- Coconut Oil, Gotu Kola herb, Ginkgo leaf, Skullcap Flowering herb, Sage herb, and Rosemary leafy tip. (Stay away from white sugar, it kills brain cells).

Breasts-4- Vitamin D, Green tea, Lycopene.

Bronchi-9- Marshmallow Root, Mullein Leaf, Chickweed Herb, Pleurisy Root, Lungwort Herb, and Lobelia Herb.

Cartilage-6 &10- Legumes, Pomegranates, White Oak Bark, Lungwort Herb, Marshmallow root, Mullein Leaf, Black Walnut Leaf, Gravel Root, Slippery Elm Bark, Wormwood Herb, Plantain Leaf, Lobelia Herb, Skullcap Herb, and Aloe Vera Gel Powder

Ear- Black Cohosh Root, Blue Cohosh Root, Blue Vervain Herb, Skullcap Herb, and Lobelia Herb.

Eyes- 3- Eyebright Herb, Prodigiosa, Bayberry Bark, Goldenseal Root, Red Raspberry Leaf, and Cayenne Pepper.

Female Organs- 8b- Squaw vine Herb, Red Raspberry Leaf, Nettle Leaf, Dandelion Leaf, Wild Yam Root, Cramp Bark, Chickweed Herb, Purple Dulse Leaf, Chaste Tree Berry, Motherwort Herb, and Ginger Root.

Gallbladder-2- Barberry Bark, Wild Yam Root, Cramp Bark, Fennel Seed, Ginger Root, Catnip Herb, and Peppermint Leaf.

Hair-4- Honey-moisturizes hair follicles and lock in shine, Cinnamon-increases blood flow (consume externally and/ or internally), spinach-nutrients and source of iron, vitamin A and C which is essential for hair growth and distributes oils throughout the scalp, Greek Yogurt-provides protein and blood flow to your scalp and strengthens hair follicles, blueberries-provides Vitamins A, B5, C, and E, stimulates hair follicles, and removes toxins from your scalp, drink plenty of water.

Heart-1- Hawthorn Berry Juice Concentrate, Lily of the Valley, and Pure Vegetable Glycerin.

Joints-6- Boswellia Extract, Turmeric Root, Hydrangea Root, Brigham Tea Herb, Yucca Root, Chaparral Leaf, Black Walnut Leaf, Nettle Leaf, Lobelia Herb, Burdock Root, Sarsaparilla Root, Wild Lettuce Herb, Valerian Root, White Willow Bark, Wormwood Herb, Cayenne Pepper, and Black Cohosh Root.

Kidneys-11- Ginger Root, Goldenseal Root, Juniper Berry, Lobelia Herb, Marshmallow Root, Parsley Root, and Uva Ursi Leaf.

Large Intestine-2- Cape Aloe, Cascara Sagrada Bark, Garlic Bulb, Senna Leaf, Ginger Root, Barberry Bark, and Cayenne Pepper

Ligaments-6 &10- Cayenne Pepper (40 M.H.U.), Wintergreen Oil, Menthol Crystals, Cinnamon Oil, Eucalyptus Oil, Valencia Orange Oil, Cajeput Oil, Spearmint Oil, Coconut Oil, Peppermint Oil, and Camphor Crystals in a base of Extra Virgin Olive Oil.

Liver- 2- Barberry bark, Yellow Dock Root, Burdock Root, and Cocolmeca

Lungs- 1&9- Marshmallow Root, Lobelia Herb, Lungwort Herb, Mullein Leaf, Pleurisy Root, and Chickweed Herb.

Lymph Nodes-5- Red Clover, Cleavers, lemon and water, Goosegrass, Maanjisthasm, Bupleurum, and Rehmannia.

Male Organs- 8a- Eleuthero Root, Sarsaparilla Root, Red Raspberry Leaf, Saw Palmetto Berry, Ginkgo Leaf, Pumpkin Seed, Damiana Leaf, Hops Flower, Dandelion Leaf, Hawthorn Berry, and Cayenne Pepper.

Mouth-2&9- Chickweed Herb

Nails-4- Calcium

Nasal Cavity-9- Eucalyptus, Cassia, Cajeput, Pure Menthol & Camphor Crystals

Nerves-7- Black Cohosh Root, Blue Cohosh Root, Blue Vervain Herb, Lobelia Herb, and Skullcap Herb

Nose-9- Peppermint Oil, and Spearmint Oil.

Pancreas-2 &3- Cedar Berry, Uva Ursi Leaf, Licorice Root, Mullein Leaf, Cayenne Pepper, and Goldenseal Root.

Pituitary Gland-3- Queen Anne's Lace Herb, Gotu Kola Herb, Ginkgo Leaf, Mullein Leaf, Oregon Grape Root, Lobelia Herb, and American Ginseng Root.

Sensory Organs-7- Basil, Beebalm, Chamomile, Heliotrope, Hyacinth, Lavender, Lemon balm, Lily, Lily-of-the-Valley, Mint, Peony, Pinks, Sage, Scented Geranium, Stock, Thyme, Violet. Chamomile, Sweet Woodruff, Creeping Thyme, and Woolly Thyme.

Skeletal Muscles-6- Ginger.

Skin-4- Shea Butter, Prickly Ash Bark, Lily of the Valley Olive Oil, Arnica, Comfrey Root, Marshmallow Root, Marigold Flower, and Beeswax.

Small Intestine-2- Cascara Sagrada Bark, Barberry Bark, Cayenne Pepper, Ginger Root, Lobelia Herb, Red Raspberry Leaf, Turkey Rhubarb Root, Fennel Seed, and Goldenseal Root.

Spinal Cord-7- Danshen, Ginkgo, Ginseng, Notoginseng, and Astragali Radix.

Spleen-5- Codonopsis, Red Ginseng, Astragalus, Atractylodes Rhizome, Licorice, Chinese Yam, and Pseudostellaria Root

Stomach-2- Cuachalalate, Catnip Herb, and Fennel Seed.

Tendons-6 &10- Cayenne Pepper, Wintergreen Oil, Cinnamon Oil, Eucalyptus Oil, Valencia Orange Oil, Cajeput Oil, Spearmint Oil, and Peppermint Oil,

Throat-9-Wild Cherry Bark, Licorice Root, Marshmallow Root, Horehound Herb, Mullein Leaf, Ginger Root, Anise Seed, and Organic Lemon Peel, in a base of Vegetable Glycerin.

Thyroids-3- Guarana Seed, Eleuthero Root, Fo-Ti Root, Gotu Kola Herb, Mullein Leaf, and Kelp Plant

Tissue-4- White Oak Bark, Lungwort Herb, Slippery Elm Bark, Marshmallow Root, Mullein Leaf, Black Walnut Leaf, Gravel Root, Wormwood Herb, Plantain Leaf, Skullcap Herb, Lobelia Herb & Aloe Vera Gel Powder

Tonsils-5- Echinacea, Pineapple extract with bromelain, Hydrastis Canadensis, Licorice Root, Wild Indigo, Sage

Uterus-8b- Goldenseal Root, Blessed Thistle Herb, Cayenne Pepper, Cramp Bark, False Unicorn Root, Ginger Root, Red Raspberry Leaf, Squaw vine Herb & Uva Ursi Leaf.

Vagina-8b- Goldenseal Root, Blessed Thistle Herb, Cayenne Pepper, Cramp Bark, False Unicorn Root, Ginger Root, Red Raspberry Leaf, Squaw vine Herb & Uva Ursi Leaf.

Veins-1- Sophora Flower, Bilberry Fruit, Ginger Root, Butcher's Broom, Gotu Kola Herb, Stone Root, Hawthorn Berry & Marshmallow Root.

Listed below are herbs that can aid in support for specific conditions in the human body; these are specific herbs I have personally used myself and recommended for my family, friends, and love ones.

Acne- Apple Cider Vinegar, Grapefruit, Turmeric, Lemon

Arthritis- Eucalyptus, Sea Moss, Cayenne Pepper (it also come in capsule form), Potassium, Turmeric, Borax

Asthma- Mullein, Black Seed Oil, Eucalyptus, Marshmallow Root, Elecampane Root, Lobelia Herb, Lungwort Herb

Allergies- Elecampane root, Elderberry, Probiotic, Butterbur, Garlic, Rosemary

Alzheimer's- Coconut Oil, Red Palm Oil, Valerian Root, Turmeric, Lemon

Autism- Chamomile, Echinacea, Garlic, Ginseng, St. John's Worth

Back Pain- Capsaicin, Lavender, Rosemary, Peppermint, Eucalyptus, Cloves, Ginger Feverfew

Bleeding- Notoginseng

Blood pressure- Flor de Manita, Black Seed Oil, Cayenne Pepper (capsules), Celery Juice, Cucumber juice, drink plenty of water.

Bone and Tissue Support- White Oak Bar, Lungwort herb, Slippery Elm Bark, Marshmallow Root, Mullein Leaf, Black Walnut Leaf, Gravel Root, Wormwood Herb, Plantain Leaf; stay away from tomatoes, especially if you are experiencing joint pain. **Cancer-** Vitamin C with bioflavonoids, Black Seed Oil, Alkaline Diet, Anamu (Guinea Hen), Pereira Bark, Soursop (Graviola), Nopal

Cataract- Eyebright Herb, Prodigiosa.

Charley Horse-

1. Drink plenty of water,
2. Eat calcium-rich foods (almonds, figs, cheese, broccoli), these foods help muscular contraction which helps the blood vessels to pump blood better.
3. Eat potassium-rich foods (bananas, melons, avocado, sweet potato), these foods help the nervous system and the function of the muscles,
4. Eat magnesium-rich goods, (beans, nuts, seeds, whole grain), these foods stabilize what is causing muscular contraction.

Cholesterol Issues- Blackseed Oil, Garlic, Cayenne Pepper (pill form is available); note a person dealing with cholesterol issues usually have an underlining heart issue thus taking Hawthorn Berry Syrup for the circulatory system is also recommended **Congestion-** boil water with sea salt and citrus fruits (lemon peels, orange peels), then inhale the steam. Turpentine can also help with chest congestion.

COVID 19- Citrus fruit Steam (boil orange peels, onion, sea salt and inhale), Vitamin C, Zinc, and Vitamin D

Depression- St. Johns Worth

Diabetes- blood detox, organ detox, Cinnamon Bark (regulate sugar), Elderberry (boost immune system), Irish Sea Moss and Bladderwrack (target digestive system), and consume herbs to support the kidney and adrenal gland,

Energy- Muscle, ginseng, eleuthero root, bee pollen, licorice root, Brigham tea herb, Gotu kola herb, ginger root, yerba mate leaf

Eczema- oatmeal and milk bath

Fever- Prickly Ash Bark, lemon, and water

Fluid Retention- Cleaver herb, Lily of the Valley

Headaches- Peppermint Oil, Turpentine

Hot Flashes- Red Clover

Kidney Stones- Lemon and water, Chana Piedra, Lymphalin, soak in Epson salt, Lily of the valley

Low Blood Platelets- Papaya extract

Prostate Health- Anamu (Guinea Hen), Pereira Bark, Soursop (Graviola), Nopal, Saw Palmetto, Beta-Sitosterol, Pygeum, Ryegrass Pollen Extract, Stinging Nettle

Seizures- Elderberry, Blue vervain, burdock root, valerian root, bugleweed, yellow dock

Sinus- Neti Pot, Brigham Tea Herb, Horseradish Root, Cayenne Pepper

Sore throat- 1-2 teaspoons of lemon or Apple Cider Vinegar followed with warm tea and honey. Also, Marshmallow Root and Licorice Root can help with a sore throat.

Stomach- Cuachalalate

Taste Buds- lemon and water mix

Tooth Abscess- Salt water rinse, Baking Soda, Oregano, Cold Compress, Fenugreek Tea, Cloves, Thyme, Hydrogen Peroxide

Toothache- Cloves, Calendula, Yarrow and Tarragon

Tooth Infection- Turmeric, Goldenseal

Tooth Decay- Oil of Oregano

Urinary tract infections (UTI)- Pure Cranberry Juice, lemon, and water, Lily of the Valley, apples, oranges, Uva Ursi (bearberry leaf), garlic, green tea, parsley tea, chamomile tea, mint tea

Weight Loss- Protein shake, Fenugreek, Blackseed Oil, mustard oil, CBD oil, Fenugreek, Cayenne Pepper, Ginger, Oregano, Caralluma Fimbriata, Turmeric, grapefruit, lemon, black pepper

I encourage everyone to research for themselves, do not just take my word for it. This book is simply a guide.

MAINTAINING A HOLISTIC LIFESTYLE

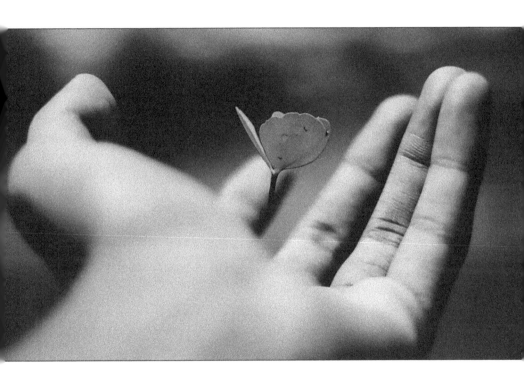

"You were running the race so well. Who has held you
back from following the truth?" (Galatians 5:7)

THE HERBS LISTED IN THE PREVIOUS SECTIONS can seem overwhelming. If you have more than one health condition, I suggest focusing on the most important conditions of your body 1st, then after experiencing healing move to the next. Sometimes too much of anything whether good or bad can be too much for your body systems and can cause a negative reaction.

Even after experiencing healing, continue to stay away from a bad diet. Keep yourself healthy, by exercising, getting the proper amount of sleep, and challenge your mind to read at least one book a day. A lack of maintaining a healthy body can cause your body to relapse and be in a worse state than before. I firmly believe that God commissions us to be a good steward of everything he has given us, and this also includes the body, our temple in which we possess. I do believe in miracles, but I also believe there are times God will meet us at the point of our need. As if God is waiting to see what we are going to do about a situation or diagnosis. In the words of Elder Tony Rainey, my assistant Pastor "do what you can and allow God to do what you can't!"

Do what is needed to build your body. Research herbs you put in your body, then evaluate yourself to see if you see a difference in any area of your life, like increased energy, sleep, focus, or memory. Remember you are in total control of what you consume. Whether that is medication or herbs!

The great thing I love about herbs is that most herbs are good for more than one thing. Thus, causing more than one area of the body to benefit and experience healing. Being a healthy individual will make you feel better physically and some cases mentally. Schedule regular checkups with your doctor to monitor your bodily progress and regular checkups will also give you a push to continue to keep going; positive progression alone is an encouragement. Reward yourself every now and then with some type of enjoyment. If you slip up on your diet, do not be too hard on yourself. Overcome it quickly and start again.

My Pastor, Richard Stampley Sr. says, "Fasting is good for you spiritually and naturally fasting gives your organs a time to rest." According to St. Matt 17:21, the spiritual benefits of fasting is the most important. Naturally, fasting detoxifies and cleanses the body from impurities, boosts cognitive performance, decreases the risk of certain diseases, protects the body from obesity and certain diseases, reduces inflammation, improves overall fitness, supports weight loss, and benefits cancer patients. Fasting has been proven to help cancer patients on chemotherapy jumpstart their immune systems. If you decide to fast for natural benefits solely, I encourage you to study various types of fasting and choose the one that is most productive for your body.

CONCLUSION

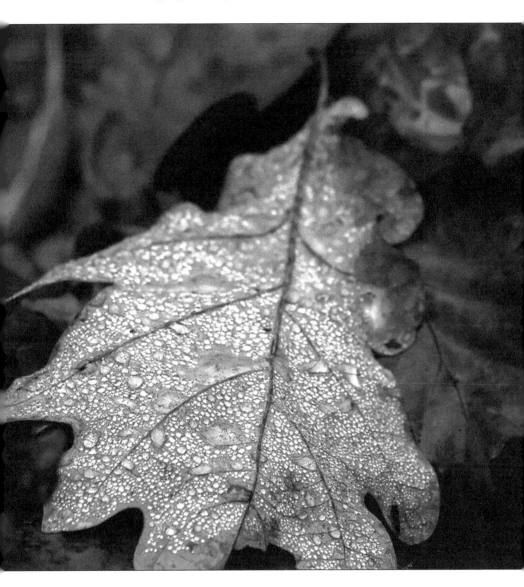

"Now all has been heard; here is the conclusion of the matter: Fear God and keep his commandments, for this is the duty of all mankind." (Ecclesiastes 12:13)

THIS BOOK IS NOT AN AVENUE OR AN EXCUSE NOT to go to a physician. I personally go to the doctor so I can get the specifics of what I need to work on within my body. In all actuality, Physicians have received years of education and knowledge about the body, so nothing is wrong with getting information from them then taking that gained information and utilizing it for healing gain. There are times I will also take the medicine to get immediate relief from certain symptoms because I know medicine pacifies the symptoms. Once completing the antibiotic and once I get the pain or symptoms under control, I wean myself off the medicine and start herbal treatment, knowing that complete healing is my ultimate goal.

I cannot cover everything in one book. My intent was to present important information so every reader will have a guide for additional research on natural healing. This book is simply a starting place. My family and I take a lot of the herbs mentioned in this book and have noticed tremendous differences within our bodies. There are many herbalists, herbs, and natural remedies for many conditions, sicknesses, and diseases we experience in our body. Read articles, books, and search to uncover the truth so you can receive true permanent healing and not a temporary relief. Dig deeper and seek answers past the symptom in which you are experiencing. You can be healthy and live a healthy long life. Retain your mind, desires, and taste buds to choose a healthier way.

Remember it is ultimately your decision of what you choose to put in your body. Remember that a lot of times when a doctor prescribes medication, and that medication does not work, your doctor will either increase the dosage or change the prescription. Doctors are practicing medicine, and it is your choice whether you allow your physical body to be an experiment or a theory. The set of explanations of a natural idea is used to account for a situation or justify a course of action. You deserve a solid justifiable understanding of everything you consume within your body.

CPSIA information can be obtained
at www.ICGtesting.com
Printed in the USA
LVHW070511020621
689027LV00021B/2268